AF855745

THE PATIENT'S LITTLE INSTRUCTION BOOK

YOUR HEALTH CARE SURVIVAL GUIDE

Carolyn Jenks *and* Gerard Spiniello

Illustrations by Darlene West Spiniello

QMP

Quality Medical Publishing, Inc.

ST. LOUIS, MISSOURI

1997

Cover art concept by Darlene West Spiniello

Printed in the United States of America.

Quality Medical Publishing, Inc.
11970 Borman Drive, Suite 222
St. Louis, Missouri 63146

ISBN 1-57626-022-4

QMP/IPC/IPC 5 4 3 2 1

To

all patients everywhere

Linda,
Keep up the good fight for all
patients everywhere.
With my high regard,
Gerry Spiriello
June 6, 1997

PREFACE

Does the medical care you are receiving measure up to the care that you had 10 years ago? If so, you are among the fortunate. Many patients in today's environment are baffled and confused by the current health care system. With new technology, the advent of managed health care, and other cost containment measures, the new medical world is complex and difficult to access and navigate. A reciprocal change in attitude and behavior on the part of patients is required. Patients can no longer afford to be passive participants in their own health care—rather, they must now become actively involved and informed consumers.

Our lifetime careers in medicine have compelled us to write this little instruction book for patients to use as a simple tool to help ensure that they receive the best care in a personal and humane way.

Carolyn Jenks, LICSW, BCD
Gerard Spiniello, PA-C

CONTENTS

Be a Student

1 Patients who take a more active, assertive, and collaborative role in their health care are more likely to have a better outcome.

2 Accepting any medical treatment on blind faith without asking questions is reckless behavior. Woe to the patient who says, "I don't want to know what you are going to do to me . . . just do it."

"The next best thing to knowing something is knowing where to find it."

Samuel Johnson

3 Most people spend more time researching and evaluating the purchase of a VCR than they do choosing a doctor, hospital, or health plan.

4 *Good* patients don't ask questions.
Good patients don't ask for explanations.
Good patients believe anything they are told.
Good patients don't want to take up a lot of time.
Good patients think everyone else is important and busy.
Good patients don't want to be a bother.
Good patients think everyone is sicker than they are.

DON'T BE A "GOOD" PATIENT.

5 Learn about the alternatives to all medical treatments, especially surgery.

6 Get a second opinion. Then get an independent third opinion.

7 Talking to a friend or relative with the same medical problem may provide emotional support, but it may not be pertinent if you are seeking medical advice. Remember, every person is different and has a unique medical history. Symptoms and treatment approaches will vary.

8 Bring a small notebook or a cassette recorder to important medical appointments. Keep these items visible at your bedside when you are in the hospital. Record information you want to tell your doctor and questions you want answered.

9 Make a practice of asking to see your medical record. You may have to submit a written request and pay clerical fees to obtain a copy. In two thirds of the states, patients have legal access to their medical records. The file in your doctor's office is your doctor's property and may be edited before it is seen.

10 *Get copies of everything!* Keep your own medical record at home in a three-ring binder. Bring it with you to all medical appointments.

11 Become a student of your medical condition.

12 If you have irritable bowel syndrome (IBS), premenstrual syndrome (PMS), chronic fatigue syndrome (CFS), or any other chronic condition, your role as a student of your medical condition is crucial. Not everyone with these frustrating problems responds to the same treatment. Trial and error may be the only way to discover what treatment works best. Time and patience are required by patient and doctor alike.

13 If you have a heart condition, ask your doctor for a copy of your latest electrocardiogram (EKG). Keep it with your important papers. *Take it with you to the hospital, especially the emergency room.* If the doctor finds no changes in the current and previous EKG, you and your HMO can be spared much time, expense, and hassle. This is especially important if you are complaining of chest pain, palpitations, or shortness of breath.

14 If you are seeking cancer information, try the Physicians Data Query (PDQ) for current information on the prognosis, staging, and treatment of cancer, as well as where clinical trials are being held. Call the cancer information service of the National Cancer Institute (NCI) at 1-800-4-CANCER (1-800-422-6237) for more information about PDQ. *Don't give up if you get a busy signal.*

15 PRACTICE PREVENTIVE MEDICINE.

16 Always ask how you could have prevented your current medical problem and how it can be avoided in the future.

17 In the early stages cancer does not cause symptoms or pain. Early detection of cancer offers the best chance for cure. Ask your doctor what cancer screening test you should have and how often. The following are suggested guidelines:

- Mammogram and clinical breast exam — every 1 to 2 years
- Breast self-exam — every month
- Rectal exam — every year
- Guaiac stool test — every year
- Sigmoidoscopy — every 3 to 5 years
- Skin exam — part of your regular health checkup
- Prostatic-specific antigen (PSA) — ask your primary care provider or urologist

18 If your doctor is going to be away, know the name of the doctor on call and how he or she can be reached.

19 In an urgent situation requiring a trip to the hospital, ask your doctor or health care provider to call the emergency room in advance.

20 Medicine is a business and the patient is a customer. Treat every medical encounter like a business relationship and demand accountability.

21 Many patients are afraid to be assertive or question their doctors, fearing they will jeopardize their care. WRONG. Being assertive and being aggressive are not the same thing. If you ask a question or state your opinion in an appropriate way, you are being assertive. You will be respected, get more time from your providers, and be more likely to be included in the decision-making process.

22 In any case of malpractice the patient must share some of the responsibility.

23 Stay assertive, alert, and involved. Once you have done your homework and selected those who will be caring for you, TRUST THEM. Don't constantly second guess your team. This will hurt your morale and theirs.

"Wherever the art of medicine is loved,
so also is there love of humanity."

Hippocrates

Doctor-Patient Relationship

24 The doctor-patient relationship is one of medicine's most powerful therapeutic tools.

25 When choosing a doctor, use your first meeting as an informational interview. Let the doctor take your history and you take the doctor's history.

26 When choosing a doctor, ask health professionals you know who they would use for their physician.

27 A doctor's reputation or notoriety is not always relevant. Find a good doctor who helps you with your problems; don't just spend your time searching for "top specialists."

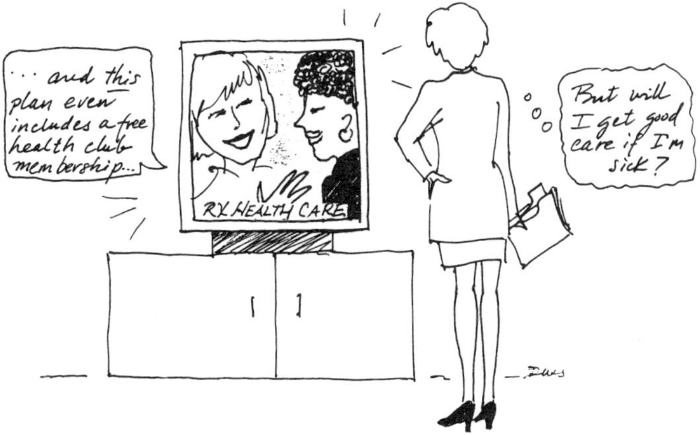

28 Physician referral services, affiliated with hospitals, are a form of advertising to promote the practices of staff physicians. These services may be an excellent starting point for getting a referral, but you need a wider choice before you make your selection.

29 Develop a relationship with one primary care provider. This ongoing relationship increases your chances of getting quality health care.

30 The most important sign of a good doctor-patient relationship is sensing you are liked as a person.

31 Studies have shown that the most important decision an AIDS patient can make is choosing the right doctor.

32 Just as you would not want a surgeon to perform an operation on you that he or she rarely does, the medical doctor who cares for you should be knowledgeable about your particular health problem.

33 Be sure your doctor is not intimidated by alternative therapies, especially if you are a cancer or AIDS patient.

34 The doctor-patient relationship must be one of mutual participation with active involvement and collaboration on the part of the patient. This kind of relationship becomes increasingly hard to maintain in the managed care environment where the industry standard requires doctors to keep office visits to 8 to 15 minutes and to see 70 patients per week.

35 The doctor-patient interaction is good if you feel:

- You *gave* accurate and complete information regarding your problem.
- You *received* accurate and complete information and answers to your questions.
- You mutually arrived at a plan of care.
- You experienced a sense of well-being.

*"One of the essential qualities
of the clinician is interest in humanity,
for the secret of the care of the patient
is in caring for the patient."*

Francis W. Peab

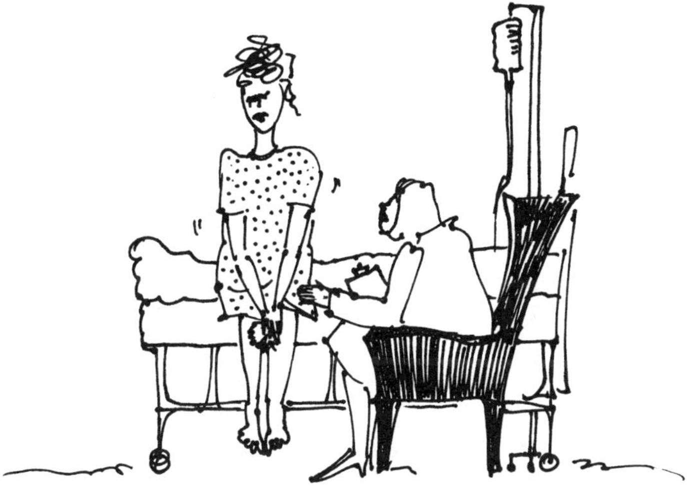

36 Good doctor-patient communication is essential to good care.

37 *Have faith.*

*"We have not lost faith,
but we have transferred it from God
to the medical profession."*

George Bernard Shaw

38 Doctors are people with the same potential for good and bad behavior as anyone else.

39 Even the very best doctors experience complications.

"I'm not sure we understand everything we know about this."

Charles M. Abernathy, Jr., M.D.

40 One of the best indicators of a doctor's competence is the ability to say, "I don't know."

41 A good doctor welcomes a second opinion.

42 *Top Ten Signs of Good Bedside Manner*

THE DOCTOR . . .

1. Sits down when talking to you (in a chair and not on your bed).
2. Makes eye contact when talking rather than flipping through your chart.
3. Doesn't act preoccupied or anxious to leave.
4. Avoids "medicalese" or asks if you understand what terms mean.
5. Inquires if someone else should be contacted to explain your condition.

6. Seems to respect you as a person and makes you feel special.
7. Ensures your privacy by closing the door or pulling the curtain, especially when discussing sensitive or highly personal information.
8. Protects your modesty during examinations by exposing only that area of the body being examined.
9. Doesn't leave abruptly if you cry or become emotional. Can deal with feelings.
10. Understands your emotional as well as your physical response to illness and is able to give appropriate support.

43 A good clinician must have more than just knowledge of medicine. Applying that knowledge to treating patients requires interpersonal skills. This combination of skills is commonly referred to as "bedside manner." Key ingredients are respect for the patient's participation, skill in communication, and patient education.

44 There is no such thing as a good doctor with a lousy bedside manner.

Your Doctor's Appointment

45 Be on time for medical appointments. Expect the same of your doctor.

46 If you insist on a particular day for a routine appointment or test, and the doctor's office agrees to "fit you in," be aware that you may have to wait and your doctor may be rushed.

47 The first step a doctor should take in solving a patient's problem is to obtain a history and perform a complete physical examination.

48 *Prepare for your doctor's appointment.*

A. Symptoms: Write down important symptoms and note the following:

• How long have they been present? • Is there anything that has aggravated or relieved these symptoms? • What have you already done to treat your condition? • What do you think might be causing these symptoms? • Have you ever had anything like this before and what helped?

B. Prior Medical History: Be prepared to discuss previous medical problems and operations. • Know the dates of operations and the names of surgeons who performed them. (This is where keeping your own home medical record comes in handy.)

C. Medications: Come prepared with a complete list of your current medications. Include dosages and number of times taken each day.

EXAMPLE: Micronase, 5 mg, once a day
Antenolol, 25 mg, twice a day
Digoxin, 0.25 mg, once a day
Lasix, 20 mg, once a day

("I take a pill for sugar, two heart pills, and a water pill" won't do.)

Or just put all the bottles in a brown paper bag and bring them with you.

D. Allergies: It is not enough to say, "I'm allergic to penicillin." Know what symptoms accompany your "reaction." Are they as simple as a mild rash or as dangerous as a life-threatening allergic reaction?

49 If you prepare for your office visit, you will have more time to talk with your provider, have your questions answered, and receive vital information. Preparedness is especially important in the age of managed care when office visits may be limited to 8 to 15 minutes.

50 If you are consulting with a specialist or getting a second opinion, bring any lab test, x-ray, or biopsy results. It is always good to bring x-rays as well as the written report. The hospital may not release the original to you, but copies can be obtained.

51 A physician is legally bound to tell a patient his or her diagnosis and prognosis unless there is good reason to believe that the patient may be harmed by the information (for example, in cases of severe depression or risk of suicide).

52 Facing an illness or surgery is stressful. No matter how organized or self-reliant you normally are, you may need help during this special time. If you have a friend or relative who can stay objective and focused, bring that person with you to medical appointments and consultations.

53 A fair question at any time is, "When can I expect to feel better?"

"It doesn't matter that everything has already been said. No one was listening."

Andre Gide

54 You have a responsibility to prevent illness by following your doctor's advice and by practicing good health maintenance and preventive medicine behaviors.

Tests

55 Avoid unnecessary tests. ALWAYS ASK . . .

- What is the purpose of this test and what information will it provide?
- How will this information be used to make a diagnosis or to initiate therapy?

Don't agree to a test unless you are satisfied with the answers to your questions.

56 When having any kind of test that will expose you to radiation, ask that your body be protected with lead shields to avoid radiation exposure.

57 Before having any test performed, feel free to ask, "When can I get the results and who will give them to me?"

58 It is okay and may even be reassuring to receive information on your test results over the phone if the news is good or routine.

59 Insist on a face-to-face meeting with your doctor to discuss any questionable test results (abnormal Pap smear or elevated PSA) or findings of a more serious nature (indicators of serious heart disease, diabetes, cancer, etc.). You should *never* be expected to receive this alarming news over the phone.

Surgery

60 When considering medical treatments, diagnostic tests, or surgical procedures, be sure that the benefits outweigh the risks.

61 New surgical procedures are constantly being developed. Make sure your doctor is experienced with the particular treatment that you have chosen.

- Ask your doctor directly, *"How many of these operations have you performed?"*
- Also ask to talk to other patients who have had this procedure.

62 Don't always insist on the newest technology. It's not necessarily the best choice for you.

63 The focus of attention should be on *you,* not the technology.

64 Good surgeons don't rush you to the operating room without considering other alternatives.

65 Ten questions to ask your surgeon if you are scheduled for an operation . . .

1. *What are the benefits and risks of this operation?*

2. *What are the potential complications?*

3. *How long does this operation usually take?*

4. *How long will I be in the hospital?*

5. *Will I lose a lot of blood?*

- This question will open a dialogue for a discussion about *autologous* blood transfusions. These are transfusions of your own blood donated beforehand for use if needed during your operation. If time permits, always try to donate *your own blood* for transfusion.

6. *What kind of anesthesia will be best?*

- Local or regional anesthesia is preferable because it numbs only that part of the body being operated on.

- If local or regional anesthesia is not appropriate, then a spinal or epidural anesthetic is the next best option. A needle or catheter (tiny tube) is placed into the space surrounding the spinal nerves and an anesthetic is intermittently or constantly infused to control pain. An epidural catheter can be left in place to provide pain relief for several days after the operation.

- If general anesthesia is necessary, you will be sedated and a plastic tube will be inserted down your throat. Anesthetic gas will be given through this tube and absorbed into your bloodstream through the lungs. The gas will keep you asleep during the operation.
- Be aware that complications increase if a general anesthetic is used. The anesthesiologist will explain the risks to you and ask you to sign a consent form.

7. *Will I leave the hospital with drains or tubes still in place? If so, how will I care for them and when will they be removed?*

8. *How long will it take for me to recuperate and resume my normal level of activity?*

9. *When can I resume sexual activity?*

10. *What is the possibility that I will die from this operation?*

- This is an appropriate time to bring up living wills and health care proxies. Let your surgeon know your desires concerning the application of extraordinary measures to prolong your life should an unexpected complication or negative outcome occur. Designate someone as your health care agent. You should also discuss any religious beliefs affecting blood transfusions and organ donation.

66 Insist on meeting with your surgeon the night before and the morning of your operation. Get answers to your last-minute questions.

67 AVOID having surgery on a *Friday* unless it is an emergency. During the weekend, staffing is lighter and caregivers may not be as available.

68 If you are having an operation on one side of your body, write WRONG SIDE in red magic marker on the other side.

69 When having a laparoscopic procedure in which a camera is inserted, ask that a videotape be made as a record.

70 The surgeon who has just performed your operation has an obligation to talk to you and your loved ones in person. Don't settle for calls from the OR locker room or the car phone.

ACCEPT NO SUBSTITUTES!

71 You, the patient, are really the one who can prevent complications after surgery. Here's how. . . . Get the hell out of bed as soon as possible. Move your legs, cough, and deep breathe every hour.

The Hospital Stay

72 *What to bring to the hospital:*

- Two large safety pins to close the curtains tightly around your bed for privacy
- Pencil and notebook
- Portable cassette player or CD player and your favorite music
- *The Patient's Little Instruction Book*

- Your daily planner or other notebook containing important phone numbers, insurance information, and a list of medications and allergies
- Reading material
- Someone who loves you

What to leave at home:

- Hostile relatives
- Anything valuable

73 When being admitted to the hospital, ask for a copy of your rights and responsibilities as a patient. Then read it.

74 Don't go to a hospital that doesn't have an ethics committee? How will you know? Ask!

75 Most hospitals have interpreter services. If English is your second language, you may want to inquire if these services are available.

76 Many hospitals are developing specific plans of care called CLINICAL PATHS that outline exactly what will happen to you during your hospital stay for a specific operation or illness. They include information on tests, medications, activity, nutrition, wound care, and hospital discharge instructions. Ask for a brochure describing this "care map."

77 NEVER sign a consent form unless you read it. Always seek appropriate information before signing any consent form for a procedure or treatment. Insist on answers to your questions.

- Do you understand what it says?
- Are you comfortable with everything it says?

Write in any special requests or conditions. Cross out or change any wording that you find objectionable.

78 When you are hospitalized, make sure you have a patient identification bracelet attached to your wrist at all times.

79 Ask if there are any patients on your hospital floor who have a similar or the same last name.

EXAMPLES:

Johnson	Falcione	Levin	Al-Kidari	Smuthers
Johnston	Fazlione	Levine	Alzinari	Smothers

If the answer is yes, ask to be switched to a different floor to avoid clerical errors which could have serious consequences.

80 A room near the nurses' station is good if you need special care. A room down the hall is usually quieter as long as it is not near the doctor's on-call room.

81 Don't tolerate unnecessary noise in the hospital. If you are being disturbed, assert your rights.

82 When you are hospitalized, become thoroughly oriented to the nursing unit.

- Find out how to use all of the gadgets, especially the nurse call light.
- Find out when the nurses change shifts. Shifts are usually divided into:
  Days: 7 AM to 3:30 PM
  Evenings: 3 PM to 11:30 PM
  Nights: 11 PM to 7:30 AM
- Anticipate your needs, such as pain medication, prior to the shift change when the nurses are busy writing up reports and completing other duties.

83 In a teaching hospital, July is the month in which fourth-year medical students become doctors.

84 In a teaching hospital you have the right to refuse examination by anyone except your own doctor — although having medical students examine you can be a positive experience.

85 As a hospitalized patient you have a RIGHT to see your doctor every day . . . and your doctor has a RESPONSIBILITY to see you every day.

86 Make the most of the brief time your doctor spends with you at your bedside. Pull out your notes and invite him or her to sit down.

87 Ask if your case is going to be discussed with other specialists at any hospital meetings or conferences such as grand rounds, tumor board, or morbidity and mortality conference. If so, ask if you can attend. Bring a tape recorder or your personal advocate.

88 Your spouse or significant other has the right to visit you in the hospital at any hour of the day or night. As long as these visits do not interfere with your care, your loved ones cannot be asked to leave. If you desire, your visitor can request a cot to spend the night.

89 Have your family stagger visits to the hospital so that someone is there for you most of the day.

90 Pain control is often a critical issue when you are in the hospital. A patient-controlled analgesia (PCA) unit is a machine that delivers a predetermined amount of medication when you press a button. You are the best judge of your level of discomfort and the PCA enables you to be in control of the amount of medication delivered.

91 Some women are more sensitive to narcotics. They should alert their caregivers to this problem and the possibility of selecting a simple oral analgesic given on a regular basis.

92 Get to know the nurses by name and tell your family who is in charge of your care.

93 Find out the name of your *primary nurse* and tell your family so that they can call and ask for your nurse by name.

94 Nutrition is one of the most important elements in treating disease. But when you are sick and nobody knows what's wrong with you, the first thing done is to place you NPO (nothing by mouth).

95 It is a truism among patients that most hospital food is bad. Food becomes very important when you are sick and have lost so much autonomy. Have family and friends bring your favorite food to the hospital. You may want to order out if you are not on a restricted diet.

96 If you are receiving antibiotics to treat an infection and you develop diarrhea, this may signal the presence of a large bowel infection. Tell someone immediately. You may have developed a condition known as *Clostridium difficile* enterocolitis (also referred to as *c-diff*). This condition develops when antibiotics have killed the "good bacteria" in the colon and the "bad bacteria" are taking over. This infection is now seen frequently in U.S. hospitals.

97 Don't be embarrassed by the loss of bodily functions when you are sick. Everybody has an "accident" once in a while.

98 Anyone providing direct care in a hospital is required to wear a hospital ID badge. Be wary of anyone without proper identification.

99 NEVER take any unfamiliar medication without a full explanation from the nurse as to what it is, who ordered it, and what it is for. Medication errors occur in hospitals every day.

100 When someone arrives at your bedside to perform a test or procedure, first find out:

- Who ordered the test or procedure? You should have been told by your doctor beforehand.
- Who is performing the procedure and has he or she done many of these?

- What are the potential complications?
- Will any drugs, dyes, or solutions be injected or applied to your skin? Let people know if you are allergic to any of these substances. Many contrast dyes injected into patients for x-rays and special invasive procedures are iodine based. If you are allergic to shellfish or iodine, you may have a severe allergic reaction to these dyes.

101 Remember, it's bad form for someone to start "setting up" to do a procedure without talking to you first.

102 Sign a consent form only after you have had all your questions answered and are satisfied with all explanations.

103 There is no such thing as a routine or minor procedure. If you are not dead on arrival, your condition can always potentially be made worse by medical treatment.

104 When a test has to be REPEATED this should send up a red flag. Find out why. If the test must be repeated because of a mistake, make sure you are not going to be charged for the second test.

105 When in the hospital, do not permit your blood to be drawn more than once unless you are given good reason why it should be taken more often.

106 If after two tries the person attempting to draw blood has not found a vein, ask to have someone else do it.

107 If you are critically ill in the intensive care unit, a special device known as a central line or arterial line can be inserted to avoid unnecessary needlesticks and damage to your veins if multiple blood samples are needed.

108 Sometimes a consultation with the hospital chaplain can be reassuring.

109 If you are hospitalized for more than a few days, begin to keep a daily journal.

110 Hospital public relations information says, "Come to us. We are a loving, caring, nurturing family." But when you get there you may realize that it is a dysfunctional family. Rude behavior on the part of the staff should not be tolerated. Although caregivers may be feeling frazzled and frustrated because of downsizing efforts which force them to do more with less, that's not your problem. It is perfectly acceptable to let your caregivers know when their behavior is upsetting to you. *Remember . . .*

YOU ARE THE PATIENT!

111 Social workers, nurses, and discharge planners may come to your bedside to visit with you to determine if you are a candidate for early release. Be aware that this is their purpose.

112 Clinical social workers in hospital settings have psychiatric training. If you agree to see them for "support," you will generate a psychiatric diagnosis in your permanent hospital record.

113 Be sure that you get adequate discharge instructions in writing before leaving the hospital. You want to obtain information on:

- Diet
- Activity (including bathing, driving, and sexual activity)
- Medications (prescriptions and instructions on how and when to take them and side effects to watch for)
- Follow-up appointments
- Telephone numbers (who to call in case of a problem)
- Special instructions (care of wounds, tubes, and drains)

114 When it's all over and you are feeling better, don't forget to thank all of the wonderful people who have been involved in your care.

Mental Health

115 Know — before you get burnt out, stressed out, or thrown out — what mental health benefits your plan covers.

116 If your HMO limits you to four or five sessions for individual psychotherapy, you may need to explore other resources for counseling, such as private practitioners who offer a sliding scale or community- or hospital-based support groups. Another source of support you might want to investigate is a twelve-step program.

117 *Top Ten Reasons To Choose A Social Worker As Your Therapist*

1. Most of them in private practice will see you for a reduced fee if money is a problem.
2. They are trained to look at the whole person (body, mind, spirit, and environment).
3. They are people-oriented professionals, which is why most of them went into this field.
4. Some of them will go to the mat for you, even risking supervisor disapproval.

5. If you are lucky, you'll find a social worker who can help you through the dark night of your soul.
6. They have empathy in spades.
7. Most of them are in therapy themselves and/or have excellent supervision.
8. They can refer to a psychiatrist for medication or a psychologist if you need tests. They know their way around most systems and bureaucracies.
9. Only an occasional one thinks he or she is God.
10. They are comfortable admitting their mistakes.

118 Consult the yearly *Diplomate Directory* of the American Board of Examiners in Clinical Social Work (ABECSW) for a list of private practitioners in your area and their credentials.

119 Twelve-step programs offer another option for help. These focused groups provide immediate peer support (no paperwork), confidentiality, anonymity, and access to community resources, all without fees. Here are just a few:

- Alcoholics Anonymous (AA)
- Family Members of Alcoholics (AlAnon)
- Overeaters Anonymous (OA), Eating Disorders (HOW)
- Gamblers Anonymous (GA)
- Debtors and Compulsive Spenders Anonymous (DA)
- Sex and Love Addicts Anonymous (S&L Anon)
- Artists Anonymous(ArtsAnon)
- Narcotics Anonymous (NA)

and many more . . .

120 "Brief therapy" is an oxymoron.

121 "Brief therapy" is the rage today because it contains mental health costs. Legions of mental health professionals are getting on the "brief treatment" bandwagon because they have no other viable alternative to enable them to continue to deliver services.

122 "Brief therapy" is the model that contains costs for insurance companies.

123 Psychotherapists today have to be creative and persistent when recommending an extended length of service for a client within the HMO.

124 This is not a good time for anyone to be clinically depressed, but oddly enough just about everyone is.

Insurance Companies / HMOs

125 Don't wait until you have a serious illness to learn the details of your health plan. Make time to study it. Just as you take time to learn how to use your computer and how to surf the Internet, take time to learn the intricacies of your HMO or your insurance policy.

126 A health plan should give you just that, a plan to help you stay healthy. This should include advice and counseling on diet, exercise, cancer screening, stress reduction, and monitoring of laboratory studies for cholesterol levels and other indicators of chronic disease.

127 Under the fee-for-service system doctors are frequently paid for doing too much. Under managed care they are often paid for doing too little.

128 Remember that the job of the person answering the phone at an HMO is to screen incoming calls. If the situation is pressing, firmly insist, "I want to speak with my doctor."

129 In the course of your medical care if you get the feeling you are being treated like a unit on an assembly line, you probably are. Let people know how you feel.

130 Clerical errors can occur in any billing system. Examine your medical bills carefully. You may find charges from doctors you never saw or for service you never received. Make sure adjustments are made.

131 Don't confuse merger mania with health care reform.

132 Remember, a primary goal of managed care is to manage cost.

133 Books written by HMO and insurance company personnel will present their point of view. Remember, as in any promotional piece, the objective is to increase business and inspire trust in the company.

134 It must be remembered that a *for-profit HMO* is a business focused on controlling the bottom line.

135 New strategies to help insurance companies save money abound. The latest buzzword is "disease management," which describes a cost-effective way to treat certain conditions or diseases by focusing on prevention rather than treatment.

136 Don't be intimidated by rules.

137 As a member of an HMO you must be an active participant in your health care. Read the HMO's instruction book if they have one. Obtain literature outlining their conditions, restrictions, rules, regulations, procedures, warnings, and guidelines. HMO members need to know how to navigate the system. For example, if you receive care at an HMO health center:

- Know where to go when the center is closed.
- Know how to get information from the center when it is closed, such as your medical record and your x-rays.
- Know where to go for medical care in an emergency.

138 In an emergency your HMO may expect you to distinguish between an "urgent-care situation" and a "life-threatening emergency." Patients don't always know what constitutes a medical emergency. Front-line personnel such as receptionists, registration clerks, and answering services also don't always know. The following are some symptoms that must not be dismissed.

• Chest pain • Shortness of breath • Sudden irregular heart rate • Sudden blindness in one eye (even if it only lasts a few minutes) • Sudden numbness or weakness in an arm or leg • Facial numbness or muscle weakness • Severe abdominal pain • Rectal bleeding • Repeated episodes of vomiting • Vomiting blood • Temperatures 103° F or above

139 If you are one of the 35 million U.S. citizens who lack health insurance, here are some strategies:

- Join together with members of any trade association or group to which you belong to get a group rate on health insurance.
- If you are self-employed, contact the small business association in your area.
- Check out small insurance companies nationwide.
- Ask your local librarian or surf the Internet web pages.

140 Even though medicine is going through a period of rapid change, America still offers the best overall medical care in the world.

Drugs / Pharmacology

141 If you are allergic to a medication, this is *very* important information.

- Know the name of the drug.
- Tell everyone who takes your medical history.
- Tell everyone who hands you a prescription or a pill.
- Have a sign placed above your hospital bed stating:
  "ALLERGIC TO ________" (fill in the blank).

142 Always know the names of any prescription medications you are taking and the dosage. Carry a complete list in your wallet or daily planner.

143 When possible, accept a generic brand of a prescription drug. It's cheaper.

144 When your health care provider writes you a prescription:

- Remind him or her of any allergy, intolerance, or chronic disease you have, such as diabetes or asthma.
- Ask about side effects you should look for.
- Remind your caregiver of medications you are already taking on a regular basis. This becomes especially important in the clinic style of care where you may see a different provider at each visit who may not know your history. It is also important for those patients seeing multiple specialists who all prescribe drugs for different problems.

145 Your pharmacist is a valuable source of information. Ask your pharmacist how a medication should be taken and if there are any special precautions.

146 Try to get all your prescriptions filled at the same pharmacy so the computer can cross-reference the medications for dangerous drug interactions.

147 A drug should be considered the last step in solving a patient's problem, never the first. The LEAST medicine is often the BEST medicine.

148 Don't insist your doctor prescribe an antibiotic for symptoms of a common cold caused by a virus. Antibiotics are only effective against bacteria. Overprescribing antibiotics has led to the development of bacteria resistant to antibiotics.

Home Health Care

149 Some patients treated in the intensive care unit 5 years ago can now be treated at home.

150 Your insurance company may expect you to have certain therapies at home. Three years ago that meant physical therapy, speech therapy, or a visiting nurse to monitor your blood pressure. Today it means feedings through tubes and central IV lines, antibiotics, and complicated dressing changes.

151 A central IV line is placed in a patient who will require long-term IV therapy at home. These lines can be left in place for long periods of time without being changed.

152 A central line inserted in the neck (internal jugular vein) or the chest (subclavian vein) carries the risk of complications of infection, vessel injury, and collapsed lung during insertion. *Ask for a PICC* (peripherally inserted central catheter). This is inserted more safely through a vein in the arm, resulting in less pain and fewer complications during insertion. It serves the same purpose for long-term IV therapy at home as a neck or chest line.

*"It's impossible
to experience one's death objectively
and still carry a tune."*

Woody Allen

Death & Dying

153 Health care proxy and living will . . .
Don't leave home without them!

- *Proxy forms* designate someone for medical decision making for you in the event that your mental functioning is impaired.
- A *living will* specifies your wishes and instructions about artificial life support and organ donation. None of this requires a lawyer.

154 The most important goal of medicine is to relieve suffering, not prolong vegetative states.

155 Try to recognize and avoid medical futility. This is when doctors continue to aggressively treat a patient who has no hope of survival or a quality existence (known as MUMBA or CHI CHI by the resident staff).

MUMBA = Feeding tube, tracheostomy, prolonged dependence on ventilator

"Hope lies in the possibility of a resistance that is based on being able to face our reality as it is."

Bell Hooks

156 One of the final choices in life is how you are going to die. Think about it, envision it, and share it with the people who can help you make it happen your way.

157 Give your doctor a "stress test" on the subject of your death. Bring up the topic and see what happens. Burst the bubble of denial.

158 There is no excuse for any patient to die in pain. If there is one thing that modern medicine has learned to do well it's how to alleviate pain. The results of a large-scale study of terminal patients recently published in the *Journal of American Medical Association* reveal that too many patients still die in pain.

"When your fear decreases
your energy increases."

Ruth Berger

159 It's a good idea to think about your own death every day. You make every day sweeter when you allow one thought to enter your consciousness at some point that reminds you of your mortality. Then say to yourself, "I have this day ahead of me," so in this way each day becomes a gift. To practice death is to practice freedom.

*"If the dying patient wants to retain
some control over the dying process,
he must get out of the hospital if he is in,
and stay out of the hospital if he is out."*

George Annas, J.D.

160 There is no place on earth where death cannot find us.

161 Whenever possible a person should die at home.

162 If you must face your final days in the hospital, significant others can do much to make you comfortable. They can bring in plants, flowers, pictures of loved ones (pets in some cases), and any other personal effects that might bring joy and comfort to you. Play your favorite music. Children may even be allowed to visit you in the hospital in those special last days.

163 Dying should be seen as a sacred process.

164 Thinking and talking about death does not make you a student of dying; it makes you a student of living.

165 No one should ever die in an intensive care unit. When a person is dying, all tests and invasive procedures should stop. You should be allowed to die in a private room without the noise of machines and personnel.

166 A peaceful death is an essential human right.

Words of Wisdom

167 Anger and anxiety are *normal* responses in patients trying to deal with illness. There is nothing to feel guilty about.

168 CANCER is *not* a death sentence.

169 Don't lose your sense of humor.

170 Quit smoking.

171 Remember that everything takes longer than you think.

172 Sometimes the smartest, kindest, most compassionate and caring people in the system don't have any letters after their names.

173 Think critically.

174 Human beings make human mistakes.

175 Experience can be a matter of doing the wrong thing a hundred times.

*"To live is to suffer.
To survive is to find meaning
in that suffering."*

Viktor Frankl

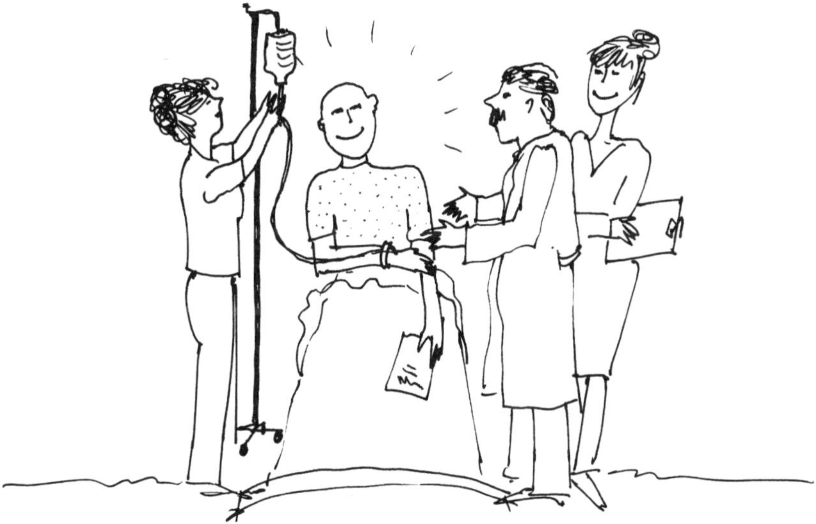

176 Always remember: As the patient *you are the center* of the health care team.

Notes

Notes

Notes

Notes

Notes

About the Authors

CAROLYN JENKS is a clinical social worker in private practice with an appointment to the professional staff of McLean Hospital in Belmont, Massachusetts, a Harvard University teaching hospital. She has worked for more than 20 years in social services and is an ardent health care reform activist.

GERARD SPINIELLO is a physician assistant in the Department of Surgery at a Harvard University teaching hospital. Over the last 20 years he has witnessed a dramatic shift in the priorities of American medicine, prompting him to take an active role in educating people about the importance of making attitudinal changes about our health care system.

If you have any insights, suggestions, or medical experiences you would like to share with us for our next book, please send them to:

The Carolyn Jenks Agency
24 Concord Avenue, Suite 412
Cambridge, MA 02138

Ordering Information

Additional copies of *The Patient's Little Instruction Book* or any of QMP's consumer health books listed below may be purchased from most booksellers, via e-mail or our home page on the Internet at qmp@qmp.com, by fax (314-878-9937), or by mailing the following order form. Substantial discounts on orders of 10 or more books are also available. For information, call Quality Medical Publishing's Special Sales Division toll-free at 1-800-348-7808.

Book Title	Price Each	No. Copies	Total Price
The Patient's Little Instruction Book ISBN: 1-57626-022-4	$10.00	________	________
A Woman's Decision: Breast Care, Treatment & Reconstruction ISBN: 1-942219-04-X	$18.50	________	________
What Women Need To Know About Breast Self-Examination ISBN: 1-942219-99-6	$1.95	________	________
What Women Want To Know About Breast Implants ISBN: 1-942219-61-9	$6.00	________	________